The Art of Meeting Your Self: Lea...
Busy World. Copyright © 2014 by

Book   ISBN 978-0-9563139-4-2

Audio ISBN 978-0-9563139-5-9

GW00372245

British Library Cataloguing in Publ...
A catalogue record for this book is available from the British Library

The right of Deborah Coote to be identified as the author of this work has been asserted by her in accordance with Copyright, Designs and Patents Act, 1988

Published by Deborah Coote, Little Ryse, Great Easton, Great Dunmow, Essex, CM6 2HD
Printed and bound in the United Kingdom by Altone Limited
www.altone.ltd.uk

Front cover photograph by John Parfrey

Book designed by CT Productions www.ctproductions.co.uk

www.deborahcoote.com

Contents

Foreword   7

Definitions   10

Introduction   12

How to use this book   14

Mindfulness Practices   17

Chapter One: Eight days a week   21

Chapter Two: The air that I breathe   27

Chapter Three: Get your socks off!   31

Chapter Four: It's the same old song   36

Chapter Five: Sitting here, resting my bones   41

Chapter Six: Comfortably numb   45

Chapter Seven: Here we are now, entertain us!   49

Chapter Eight: Let go of your heart, let go of your
                  head, and feel it now   54

The last word   58

Acknowledgements   60

Recommended Reading   61

Useful Information   62

More Books and CDs by Deborah Coote   63 *for John*

Foreword

This book nearly never saw the light of day. During the last few years, I've been temporarily dislodged by the big three (death, divorce, moving house), which meant that producing a roast dinner was an uphill struggle, let alone another book. But then, it's all about timing.

A few months ago, my friend Jane asked me if I'd speak about my work to a large fledgling group in London who are interested in mindfulness. She updated me by saying how "mindfulness" was sweeping the City, bringing with it an interest in wanting to know more.

I groaned inwardly before preparing to say "no", sincerely hoping it wouldn't be just another fad. I've been running meditation workshops and retreats alongside the Alexander Technique for individuals and groups for over a decade, having scaled down the number and frequency. Jane has been a regular attendee at several of these events, and when I think back to that first meeting with her looking like a rabbit in the headlights, Jane's self-transformation has been quite something.

Any reluctance about going back to my former working environment quickly evaporated as Jane explained about her group, and how they'd look forward to hearing my observations and insights. If she believed I had something interesting to share with her colleagues and fellow employees, then perhaps it *was* time to say it out loud. My groups and workshops have beneficial and often unexpected effects on those people who attend. And so, I changed my mind.

Timing ... it is May, 2014. I am in Sardinia, celebrating my birthday, finally writing this book, and relieved to release it from my cells. Over the years, I've had the privilege to walk alongside hundreds of people who uncover ways to wellness by living mindfully, using principles integral to the Alexander Technique and meditation. This book is about those people.

There comes a moment when you know your life is in your hands. Finding the means whereby is the challenge. Once you discover your own path, reclaiming your Self is the only possible outcome. It's impossible to give your best if you are run down, exhausted or apathetic. The art of meeting your Self with an absence of guilt, and with a selfishness that is ultimately unselfish, is worth investigating.

This is your moment.

Definitions

Self

The word 'Self' is used throughout the book. This is a familiar word in our vocabulary. Don't we already know what it means? Yes, of course we do, but in this book it has a special meaning.

F.M. Alexander (1869-1955), who founded the Alexander Technique over one hundred years ago, used the term 'Self' deliberately as a way of illustrating the mind-body connection. Self refers to the wholeness of a person, in the sense of a unified being in whom mind and body are inseparable. Alexander was well aware even back then that the accepted view was of mind-body division, the mind over matter. He was a man ahead of his time because he challenged the idea that the mind and body operated separately.

There is still a tendency in our culture to accept

without question that if we control the mind, the body will tough it out, no matter what. Ever heard the expression 'stiff upper lip?'

Mindfulness

The Oxford English Dictionary gives the following definition of ***mindfulness***:

'a mental state achieved by focusing one's awareness on the present moment, while calmly acknowledging and accepting one's thoughts, feelings and bodily sensations, used as a therapeutic technique'.

In this book the word ***mindfulness*** is used with the same meaning as given in the dictionary citation.

Direction

In the Alexander Technique, "directions" are messages from the brain to the muscles via the nerves. They help to stop us doing too much, too soon, or prevent us from doing things badly.

Introduction

The purpose of this book is to share the experiences and journeys that hundreds of my students are taking: They, like me, are learning to consciously look after themselves mindfully, with a kindness that is unfamiliar in our culture. Reading it may mark a turning point in your life. Unlearning lifetime habits of effort, excess tension, judgement and self-criticism can be challenging, especially as we don't yet live in a culture that celebrates authentic behaviour. Most of what you read in this book is common sense and may well be familiar: things you already know but may have forgotten.

Learning to live mindfully in this busy world is the most exciting and courageous thing you can undertake. It becomes a quest initially. You may uncover aspects of your character and nature you don't like, or no longer serve you well. You may be surprised when you find out how your tensions are created. Just by simply becoming aware, by witnessing rather than judging what you find, your Self will, subtly, organically, let go of the unwanted stresses and strains, softening your edges, revealing your authentic, healthy, loving Self, which is strength, not a weakness. It takes time, but where's the fire? It's also much easier than you think.

Don't watch your life from the side-lines...it's time to jump right in!

"There's only one corner of the universe you can be certain of improving, and that's your own Self"
Aldous Huxley

How to use this book

"The Art of Meeting Your Self: Learning to Live Mindfully in a Busy World" is a practical book. It's also a little book for good reason. There is so much to say on this subject that there was a risk of it becoming a War and Peace! I have to remind myself less is definitely more especially as everyone is busy! There are mountains of inspirational works out there for you to discover, should you feel inspired to do so. Once you open the door to your own treasure trove, however, you may not need to look elsewhere.

This is not an Alexander Technique book. Nor is it a book about meditation. It is neither, and yet it is both, as the experience gathered over the years has largely come from my work with people in these two arenas. You'll find a full description of the Alexander Technique and Meditation on page 17. For information on books that show you how to meditate, or books about the

Alexander Technique, see page 61 Recommended Reading.

This book is written with a light touch, giving you space and time to breathe. After all, life isn't meant to be taken so seriously is it? There are no exercises, no homework and no rules to follow. This echoes and reflects one of the basic tenets of AT, which urges students and teachers not to constantly nag themselves with 'must do this' and 'should do that' running commentaries. Such phrases are unhelpful.

At the end of each chapter you'll find a suggestion or two which may chime in with your way of thinking. If so, try them out.

The CD that accompanies this book can be used independently.

❖ Track One, *Inhabiting your Mind-Body* is a guided body awareness meditation

❖ Track Two, *The Body Breathes Itself*, focuses on the breath. It is calming and creates an anchor into the present moment

❖ Track Three, *An Abundance of Wellness*, is a guided visualisation in which you appreciate feeling well.

Mindfulness Practices:

Meditation, the Alexander Technique and Lying Down in semi-supine

Meditation is one of the methods used in mindfulness work. It isn't about escaping, controlling or stopping thought. In Tibetan Buddhism, the word "meditation" means to become familiar. It's about knowing the nature of your own mind, what type of thoughts you have, skillful and unskillful, and bringing awareness to the whole process of thinking.

There are hundreds, perhaps thousands of different types of meditative practices and methods, depending on culture, religion and personal preference, ranging from body awareness and breathing, to using mantra and transcendental methods.

The Alexander Technique is a mind-body method

that helps you to take conscious control of your Self, no matter what you are doing. By working with a teacher on a one-to-one basis, you learn to direct your thinking in activity, so that you move without unnecessary tension, effort and strain.

By stopping before taking action, and directing your thinking, you unlearn unconscious habits, allowing the body to move more naturally. The "directions" are thoughts sent to the body via the nervous system: they are not things to do, such as stretches, pushes or pulls. Examples of directed thinking may include freeing the neck, lengthening the spine, and widening the back. After a while, movement generally becomes freer, lighter and easier.

The Alexander Technique was discovered by F.M. Alexander over one hundred years ago. It attracts people of all ages and from all walks of life.

Lying Down in semi-supine

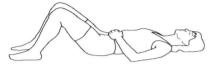

Bringing the mind and body together when lying down will help you to recognise and release muscular tension, and cultivate mindfulness.

It is important to lie on a firm surface, with your knees bent, in line with your hips, and your hands resting on your abdomen.

Place some books under your head, at the back of your skull, so that the back of your neck is unobstructed. Make sure that your head is not pushed too far back or too far forward, as this will restrict your breathing. Keep your eyes open during the session. Think about your weight being evenly distributed between the back of your head, your shoulder blades, your lower back and your feet.

While you are lying in this semi-supine position, you can think about the following directions. It is important not to try to "do" them – just use your thinking to bring about the changes.

- ❖ Allow your head to sink back into the books
- ❖ Let your body release to the floor
- ❖ Think of your spine lengthening and your back widening
- ❖ Think about your knees pointing up to the ceiling

When you get up, you can try to maintain this awareness of your Self as you go about your daily activities.

Chapter One
Eight days a week

When did we get so busy? The world has gone a bit bonkers, hasn't it? Just believing our behaviour is normal shows how much we've lost our way. This extreme busyness may be traced back to the industrial revolution, or to widespread education, to increased technological advance and labour saving devices. Who really knows? The back-story may be interesting to social historians, but how does that help us to say "no" to persistently working late, or saying "yes" to genuine offers of help? When I think of what I used to cram into my week it beggars belief. My body stopped me in the end: for some people it's the mind that gives way. Whatever it is, your Self will know how to stop you in your tracks.

For all society's obsession with our health and safety, mental health at work initiatives, wellness, ergonomic and fitness regimes, the numbers of musculoskeletal issues, stress and psychological problems are on the increase. We are clearly not very well. And yet, here in the West, having exhausted our appetites for all things materialistic, we are now embracing Eastern contemplative methods like mindfulness, while our friends in the East are cranking up production. It's a funny old world!

Practically speaking, if you are contemplating a life of mindfulness, it may help you to know exactly where your hip joints are, and how to prevent your head pulling down and contracting your spine, especially if you have a bad back or poor posture. It's really hard to maintain a good yoga asana, meditation position, or T'ai chi pose when your body bends in the wrong way. This is one reason why the Alexander Technique is useful as a mindfulness practice, although it is in, and of itself, mindful. There is something quite magical about moving well, no matter where you are or what you may be doing.

Perhaps it's time to stop, and lie down in semi-supine. One of the most common laments from my students is trying to find between ten and twenty minutes in their day to stop and lie down (full description on page 17), and yet, have no problems sitting in front of the telly or laptop for hours. Bear in mind that many people coming for the Alexander Technique have some kind of musculoskeletal issue, no matter what background they come from. Lying down is one of those simple, effective things to use as, in a non-doing way, it brings the mind-body back together. It's totally mindful. It also allows the spine to decompress, taking pressure off the inverterbral discs, allowing the spine to lengthen, and alleviating acute and chronic back pain, poor breathing and stress.

So why is it so hard to find the time? A recent conversation with a pupil with chronic back pain went something like this:

"Hello Simon. How's your Alexander week been?"

"Not great" (looks sheepish)

"How much lying down have you managed?"(Trying not to sound like a sergeant major on inspection!)

"Only once...I promised to decorate my son's bedroom, and then I was helping install central heating so I had to move a heavy radiator..."

No mindfulness there yet! However, for every one person who doesn't manage to stop and rest occasionally, there are many who do, reaping huge health benefits for very little expenditure.

So, life is busy. Take some time out. Take a lunch break. Move your body. Look at different scenery. It enlivens the mind, switching you on in a skilful, creative way. When you get home, ignore the post and phone messages, let the dog in the garden and lie down, somewhere quiet from anywhere between ten and twenty minutes, a few times a week, especially after exercise or decorating your kids' bedroom. The results will be unexpected. If life is okay, try lying down anyway. Effortless. Non-doing. No brainer!

Mind-body, body-mind ... they don't function separately. Every thought you have either finds itself via the brain to the muscles or the glandular system (think of someone you fancy then check the physical effects on your body. Then think of someone who winds you up...!)

Learning to spot that moment when tension arrives, and deciding if it is appropriate, is a skill worth developing. When the body-mind is in communication, it's easier to stay connected to your Self, remaining in that state of awareness for longer periods as time goes on. Anything that can help you be mindful of these processes is really useful. And guess what, you are the only person who can do this!

❖ *Track one on the CD, Inhabiting your Mind-Body, guides you through body awareness. Try it lying down or sitting upright in a chair, with your feet in contact with the ground*

Chapter Two
The air that I breathe

The breath is a funny old thing. If we had to remember to switch it on, we'd have dropped dead years ago! Taking a breath is the first and last thing we do in life; it links each moment from birth to death, binding every experience in between. And yet, we either take it for granted, we interfere with its natural functioning, or we make it go to places in the body it really doesn't want to go to. Ask any opera singer!

The word "inspiration" is an old French Latin word meaning breathing in, inhalation. When you sit at your computer or laptop, take a long drive, or sit in front of the telly for hours, your breathing may become shallow. This leads to a lack of oxygen in your brain (the place where you need it most at that moment), and in your body. How can you hope to be "inspired" under these circumstances?

In my world, the body breathes itself. There is nothing to do but get out of your own way and allow the breath to work. It's classic in non-doing. One of F.M. Alexander's greatest insights was the less we interfere with the natural functioning of the breath, the better it serves us. He also discovered that an excess of tension in the body, particularly around the neck and rib cage, prevents the lungs from working well as it diminishes the space required for efficient breathing.

Lots of things tighten us up. Most of us occasionally hold our breath. Life can sometimes feel like an emergency. Whatever is happening, take the opportunity to gently breathe out. No need to strain, or count. Just breathe out as if you were gently blowing a candle, trying to keep the flame alight. At the end of the out-breath, close your lips, and observe your breath naturally coming back into your body through your nose, without interfering with it. Try not to sniff, or gasp. Simply be a witness to your breath, coming and going, ebbing and flowing.

That's it. Nothing more, nothing less.

You can try this at your desk, in the car, when the train is delayed, before a meeting or presentation or when the kids are playing up. Breathing out immediately dampens down the part of the nervous system which deals with stress and tension. A fresh, natural in-breath revitalises all your systems, in fact, every cell in your mind-body. So, take just a few out-breaths every now and again. Remember, less is more, it's not an exercise. Just take one or two conscious out and in breaths, here and there.

The breath also anchors you to the here and now. When you breathe well, you feel well. It's impossible to attend to your breath consciously while simultaneously thinking about the past or future, (what you should have said to so-and-so last week, what you are going to do next week). In almost every meditative tradition, attention to the breath is regularly encouraged and practised. This is not new: it really works!

❖ *Track Two on the CD, Your Body Breathes Itself,*
guides you through a meditation on the breath

Chapter Three
Get your socks off!

Feet are truly amazing! Carrying us through every single adventure in life, our feet are another of our unsung heroes in need of acknowledging. Inhabiting the southern region of the body, our feet can however, feel a bit neglected. After all, the fun is happening up north where the senses are. Feet are such an important and underrated part of the Self, and yet, unless we feel pain or discomfort, or require a certain type of running shoe, they are often taken for granted.

When you sit down, do you ever notice your feet? For instance, do you know what your feet are up to when you are at your desk, or sitting at the breakfast table? Are they in contact with the ground, or are they twisted around your chair, or tucked back so that your feet are off the ground completely?

From an energy and effort perspective, when your feet are in full contact with the ground, it's easier for your body to be balanced. It's also efficient, costing very little energy. As soon as your feet lose contact, other parts of the body, usually in the lower back, have to tighten up to stop your body from falling. That's bad news if you suffer with back ache.

A good few years ago Mark came to see me as he was suffering from a bad back, stress and general fatigue. I knew he had a science background as his wife who bought him the lesson as a gift was also in the same field of work. I expected a healthy dose of scepticism along with lots of questions and wasn't disappointed as it makes for an interesting and lively lesson (he confessed much later to me that at the time, he thought I was bonkers).

At the end of the lesson, I asked Mark if he noticed how much his feet moved: that they were moving around throughout the entire time he was there. Talk about nervous tension and wasted energy! He said he hadn't noticed, he thanked me and left. You can imagine my surprise when Mark called a fortnight later to book a series of lessons. He said that he'd been watching his feet ever since the lesson, and that if they were doing that without him knowing, what else might he be doing to himself that was wasting his energy? This was a challenge he couldn't resist.

Six years on, everything has changed. By giving himself permission to stop and look at his unconscious responses to various things coming his way, and to his habitual ways of moving, Mark is able to pause and take a breath, to free his neck of tension. This has enabled him to reduce his stresses and strains, giving his mind-body sufficient time, energy and know-how to stay well. This is a good example of Alexander's principles of 'directing' which was mentioned on the Definitions page.

Feet have to read the terrain, which is more of a

challenge in shoes. Few of us stand in an upright, balanced way. Look at your shoes: every shoe tells a story. You may lean left, right, on your heels or on your toes. The more tension in the bones, muscles and tendons of the feet, the more difficult it is for your brain to pass information through your nervous system and back again to your body, so that you know exactly where you are in space. Only then is your body able to make the appropriate adjustments to your balance and coordination.

A good friend of mine, Sharon, is either out and about, or has her head in a book. I suggested she venture out into her garden, no socks, and simply stand on the grass, feeling the sensations in her feet. It's an incredibly evocative thing, standing or walking across grass barefoot. It takes me right back to being seven years old again.

Similarly, on the beach here in Sardinia, walking along the water's edge, noticing the texture of the sand, the temperature of the water, the waves tickling my toes, my feet and I are content, restful and present (by the way, sunny Sardinia it ain't: we've had five days of rain and cloud!)

Whether it's in the garden, at the beach, at the coffee machine, in front of a group, or at the school gates, try standing equally on both feet, your body weight distributed between the heels and pads of the toes. You'll instantly reduce effort, waste less energy being upright and your body will feel balanced.

Taking your attention to your feet immediately brings you right back to your Self, mind and body. In times of tension or stress, when you become aware of your feet, it helps to keep you grounded and anchored. Performers, whether acting, singing or presenting do a much better job when they inhabit their feet.

Just think, you have a whole planet right beneath them – there is no way you can fall!

Chapter Four
It's the same old song

We are united by habit. No matter what culture, conditioning or background, we share the nature of the habitual. They are universal constants in our lives, keeping everything familiar and safe. Whether it's something like crossing legs and arms, twitching fingers and toes, finishing off other people's sentences, having to catch the same train, or drinking tea the same time every day, most of the time these habits are unconscious. Some habits are, of course, conscious, and not all habits are harmful.

Physical habits are easier to spot than mental and emotional habits. Have you ever noticed how you eat or drink? Not just whether it's too fast or too slow, but whether you bring your meal to your head or your head to your meal? Have you ever noticed in Asian culture, the bowl is taken up to the head? It's much better for the spine, for the digestion and for keeping your shirt clean!

While you are cultivating mindful eating and drinking, don't forget how you use your mobile phone. I watch in horror the distorted shapes of my fellow humans as they talk or text with heads habitually collapsing over their chests and pulling their spines out of shape. As I remind my nephews, phone up to heads, boys!

Habits of doing are one thing. Habits of thinking are another challenge. In one of the meditation classes the other day, Anna was telling us about her week, and heard herself say:

"I've noticed recently I seem to worry about most things, and I can feel tension rising up through my feet, travelling up into the whole of my body when I sit down to meditate. I think I must be like this all the time."

The rest of the group smiled as we agreed we are in the same boat. We all share habits of thinking, to a greater or lesser extent, that create unnecessary tension. But more importantly, this is how we define ourselves. In Anna's case, she sees herself as a "worrier". By being aware of her habit to worry, Anna can change it if she wants.

Most people that come to workshops or classes are looking for ways to change their existing state of mind-body health but struggle to do the work. You see, most of us say we want to be different but that would mean changing, and habits are hard to break. It requires time and patience, as fundamental change doesn't always happen overnight. In our quick fix, sound-bite society this is a great challenge.

Knowing a little about the nature of the brain can help to understand how we can change it. Not so long ago, scientists discovered the neuroplasticity of the brain. This means that the brain is able to remap and remould itself, firing and hard wiring new neurons with new knowledge, throughout our entire lives. The scientists no longer believe that learning / unlearning stops at a certain age. So, with repetition, we can rewire the brain, and change habits, permanently.

So, to get back to crossing legs and arms, if you want to waste energy and effort holding your limbs across your body, tightening your chest, restricting your breath, displacing your joints and generally speeding up wear and tear, go right ahead! On the other hand, when the habit comes, notice it without frustration or judgement, and reposition yourself. It's a bit like training a puppy - patience is required. Just think of those millions of happy neurons!

And while you may not be inclined to go through a Japanese tea ceremony the next time you drink your tea, observe with interest how your hands fold around your cup. Feel the texture of it, the temperature, and the shape. As you take a drink, remember you are learning the art of meeting your Self. As you lift the cup to your mouth, be aware of your spine lengthening into the space above your head, with your feet in full contact with the ground.

Most of all enjoy it!

Chapter Five
Sitting here, resting my bones

When I attended my first meditation class at a local Buddhist centre, it was agony. I couldn't sit on the cushions as my back wasn't able to support itself in an upright position. I'd been experiencing back pain in ever-increasing bouts, with temporary relief provided by the osteopath.

During the tea break I saw a poster that said something like "having trouble with your sitting posture? Try the Alexander Technique. Sign up for the next workshop". As I'd never heard of the Technique before, I made a note of the phone number in order to book on the workshop. Intrigued and anxious to find out more, the next day I signed up for the workshop, and quickly followed that by having a series of one to one lessons. Sure enough, given time, I was able to sit on the cushions for half an hour without collapsing in a heap, and I began to learn how to prevent much of the pain reoccurring.

When you are sitting, take your attention into your spine. Use the back of the chair, or cushions as support. Make sure your feet are in full contact with the ground. Think about your neck being free and relaxed (it's a bit like releasing the handbrake in the car), with your next thought to lengthen your spine. We call these thoughts "directions" as I have mentioned before.

You may already know this, but don't sit for too long. Everything stiffens up: your internal organs become sluggish and energy gets blocked. Pay your Self the attention you deserve by moving regularly, even if it's just standing and sitting. Researching my last book about meditation on the web, almost all the images I found were of sitting postures in the lotus position, hands outstretched – for a nation that doesn't squat, it's most off-putting! You may therefore be pleased to read that in my workshops and retreats, we generally sit on chairs, and occasionally lie on the floor.

In Suzuki Roshi's book, "*Zen Mind, Beginners Mind*", he describes sitting naturally for meditation in this way,

"You should not be tilted sideways, backwards or forwards. You should be sitting straight up as if you were supporting the sky with your head".

When the head is balanced freely on top of the spine, the spine is naturally straight, the back naturally widens. The heart and lungs have space to work. Breathing and circulation are no longer compromised by a body that collapses or slumps. Consequently, the brain is more alert, one of the reasons for meditating.

Please, take time to rest your bones. During my Alexander training, one of my teachers used to say "don't stand when you can sit, don't sit when you can lie down". I've never forgotten these wise words even though I struggle to apply them as often as I'd like.

Learning to direct your body effortlessly into an upright position, or semi-supine position, whether in meditation, yoga, desk-work or walking the dog, is truly mindful.

❖ *Don't forget to listen to Track One, Inhabiting the Mind-Body on the CD, guiding you into body awareness with directed thinking*

Chapter Six
Comfortably Numb

In our culture, we seem to have successfully desensitised ourselves to nearly everything, to the point where our senses are almost switched off. Glazed eyes, fixed stare; our attention spans are woefully short.

iPods, mobiles and inane chatter conspire to keep out the glory of birdsong; sunglasses, small screens, and visual overload veil our eyes from spectacular sunsets; "product", man-made fragrances, factor 50, and neoprene mask the scent of the rose; additives, fast food, mouthwash, cravings and bad language dampen down taste buds; busy hands, painted nails and ambivalence are barriers to tenderness; lack of balance, nervous system meltdown, contraction and tight necks block feelings of lightness.

Sorry for sounding so uncompromising but what I'm saying is that we need as a society to recognise the state we're in. The over-worked sensory system works its hardest to give us the best in surround sound, and here we are, more often than not, unwittingly unplugged to one of nature's marvels.

Here in Sardinia, in our Garden of Eden, the air is grey with drizzle, thunder drum-rolling across the skies, providing a sharp contrast to the surrounding colourful landscape. A cacophony of birds; sparrows, finches, swifts, blackbirds, seagulls, sky larks and martins swoop and dive, entertaining us every morning with the loudest dawn chorus in memory; African marigolds, strangely shaped cacti sprouting yellow buds, vermilion begonias, dark pink petunias, violet bougainvillea and lobelia each adding a shock of paint to the deep green grass canvas; a honeysuckle scent wafts softly through the damp atmosphere, tickling our noses with a delicate perfume as it mixes with the salty sea air, while olive and bay trees link arms with the lemon tree, her bitter lemon fruit adding a tangy flavour to our frosted glasses of iced tea.

So much for my lyrical holiday update ... senses ready and reporting for duty!

And yet, I'll bet you too have experienced many times when you've inhabited your senses fully. A shock will generally do the trick, because it can heighten emotional awareness. Remember where you were, what you were doing, how you were feeling on 9/11? How about a brand new experience, like becoming a parent, or scoring a goal, or making love – guaranteed to bring you into the present moment if you truly are there for the other. Perhaps a holiday in Sardinia or the first cool drink on a hot day will tickle the taste buds back to life, as will a walk in beautiful surroundings or the death of someone precious.

Being in your senses is much simpler than having to experience any or all of the aforementioned as a prerequisite. When you drive your car later today, pause awhile before switching on the ignition: feel the grip of your hands on the steering wheel, the balance of your head on your neck. If you notice tension, soften your hands and drop your shoulders. Keep the radio on "off" to hear what sounds are around you.

Take a moment to look at the landscape, urban, suburban, or rural, it doesn't matter where you are. You may be surprised at what you see. Feel the clothes on your body; take a long out-breath.

If you are on the train or tube, look for unnecessary tension in your body to release, stay with your breath, feel space around you, even if there is a lack of it. Remain present and remember your Self: your journey home will be different.

Mindful. Wonderful.

Welcome to the world!

Chapter Seven
Here we are now, entertain us!

Isn't technology fab? I've just got used to using a satnav, having stubbornly resisted for years for some incomprehensible reason I no longer recall. I used to set off for unfamiliar places at least an hour earlier to give myself time to "get lost". I'm laughing at my former Self as I write this, as now there is unbounded gratitude for "Dizzy": she not only gets me where I need to be with no fuss, but has also given me a better sense of direction as well as increasing my confidence on the road!

Add to the list a Kindle, an iPhone and a tablet, a majestic display of genius! Far from being distracted with all this lovely technology, it's interesting to observe just how invidious it can become if allowed. Being watchful is the key. We are so used to distracting ourselves without even realising. What do you think it is we don't want to see?

Although I am plugged in, I don't Tweet, Face book or hook up to any other social networking. It's much more rewarding to see people over a cup of tea, or in gatherings. Breaking bread together is guaranteed to de-stress a family as the everyday "stuff" gets resolved around the dinner table. It's a tragedy we don't realise what a serious effect the erosion of such an important social ritual is having on us as human beings. Of course, there have also to be times when everything gets switched off to give the Self and others a rest.

Something to consider: when you aren't being entertained by someone or something else, plug your Self into the silence that is just waiting for you to hear it. There is nothing more uplifting than being immersed in stillness, and quietness. It's out of this silence creativity is born.

Just think of the Eureka moment: insight is revealed when the brain takes a break. Drop Shakespeare and write your own sonnets. Paint your own masterpieces. Sing your own songs. Unleash your own creativeness! Everything I've ever been inspired to write or record has come from a deep restfulness either on retreat, or walking the dogs, or time spent in nature, enveloped in silence. A relaxing bath may give you an aha! moment just like Archimedes, so try that too!

In a recent class, we were talking about the power of silence, and how interesting it might be to give it a go, switching off the radio in the car, or at home as an experiment. The following week, John told us how difficult he found it, as the act of switching on the dial had become so habitual that before he was aware, the sounds of his favourite heavy metal music filled his car, to and from work.

John did, however, persevere, and shared with us the following week that he'd tried periods of silence in the car. He said he felt less wired by the time he got home. John still listens occasionally to his music, and has mixed up the heavy metal with more restful sounds. Interestingly, he says he is much more aware of the habit of hearing rather than wanting to listen.

I am sure you know what it means to enjoy the quiet. After all, most people have experienced the type of holiday that recharges and reenergises the mind-body. Who doesn't like to go to the sea, or the mountains for their summer break? The trouble is, we can't afford to wait until then. Our nervous and immune systems are crashing under the weight of all this stimulus and noise, so much so that we become afraid to be quiet. We don't unplug. We don't switch the phone off. We are becoming more and more desensitised to ourselves and our beautiful planet.

Please, be mindful and take a lunch break. There is always somewhere green to sit, especially if you work near a park or a river. Nurture your Self – it will pay you back in spades. Take that break you so seriously need. Leave the vacuuming until tomorrow. Go walk the dog without the iPod. Look around. Listen to the birds. Feel the breeze. Feel the silence underneath it all. Be brave! Take an out-breath and enjoy the freshness of the in-breath. I promise that you *will* be changed by it. If not, don't ask for your money back!

Chapter Eight
Let go of your heart. Let go of your head...
and feel it now

There's a scene in Sam Mendez's film "American Beauty" where a young man called Ricky is watching a film he made of a white plastic bag dancing on the wind. He describes this experience as being totally overwhelming, saying there is so much beauty in the world he can't take it in.

Subtly, as old patterns of tension release themselves gradually from your nervous and immune systems, it gets easier to feel the world around you. You learn to enjoy letting go, to release mind-body tensions. It feels natural, like a sigh of relief.

Although I love a glass of Merlot, the times of needing a drink to let go of my head are long gone. These days, so much is uplifting: walking my dogs, a cup of tea with friends, a good sob at the telly, dancing around the kitchen table, watching the seasons change and, of course, music (thank goodness for the totally inspirational lyrics of David Gray, Kate Bush, The Stones and Richard Thompson ... have you ever heard "1952 Vincent Black Lightening?")

It's always the simple things that matter, but we get lost in the dramas and busyness of our lives. We shut down our feeling and emotional systems so that letting go of the build-up of tensions often requires help by one substance or another. Addictions take many forms: cycling and running are as addictive as soap operas and red wine, although running in a mindful manner can be uplifting. A woman told me recently at one of the workshops that running in nature was her church. How about that!

Help is never far away. Psychoneuroimmunology, the study of the interaction between immune system function, physiology and psychology amongst other things, explains much about the increase of mind-body illnesses. Conditions such as fibromyalgia, chronic fatigue and IBS are on the increase. We clearly are able to worry ourselves into ill health. However, when you choose to tune into your Self, fully inhabiting your senses, you'll hear what your body is trying to tell you. After all, what is a gut feeling?

Nowadays we know so much about what we should eat, how much exercise and rest we should have, what our muscle to fat ratios are and so it goes on. Seventy plus years ago we were all on war rations. Look at us now, clinically obese, worrying whether to spread butter or margarine on the toast!

The Buddhist philosophy talks about the middle way. That sounds like a practical common sense approach, alongside the saying, "a little bit of what you fancy does you good". Back in the day I'd walk miles for an organic banana - thank goodness that's dropped out of the cells! My Self knows what it likes and dislikes.

There is an intelligence that works when I stop fretting and allow it. I also have a tremendous gratitude for all food, especially if it's been cooked by someone else.

Whether it's through techniques like the Alexander Technique, mindfulness practices like meditation, T'ai chi or yoga, laughing or dancing, thankfully there are many ways to encourage the Self to be mindful.

When you feel the connection between the outer world and your inner world, you are relaxed, rested and well. Allow your Self to be moved by all of life's happenings. Be present to that experience. You've earned it!

❖ *Track Three, An Abundance of Wellness, is a guided meditation into appreciating your health and wellbeing*

The last word...

Learning to meet your Self is no longer a luxury: it has become a matter of survival. As individuals who make up our world, perhaps it is time to reclaim our selves in the most skilful ways we can, and live intelligently together.

Can you imagine the subsequent changes in society and our planet then? Can we show that same loving attention to ourselves in the same way we do with children, pets, or the beloved motorbike without embarrassment or ego? We all have the potential. We all want to be well.

It really doesn't matter where the inspiration comes from to get started: the fresh Eastern breeze of mindfulness sweeping across our harsh, Western landscape is most welcome, and needed.

And so, thank you for taking precious moments to read the little book with a big heart. My wish is that something in it has resonated, or reminded you that *You* definitely are worth thinking about!

May your journey back to your Self be joyful!

Acknowledgments

To Jane Daniels, for that precious invitation, for your unbounded enthusiasm and for proving that transformation really *is* possible. Thanks to Sandra Waller, John Rowland, Kirstie Richardson, Linsey Wass and Susie Keen for reading, reviewing and giving the thumbs up to the manuscript, and to this project. Thanks also to Chris Latham for his lovely cover and book design. Huge thanks to Caroline Laidlaw for helping me to shape and refine the book. Lastly, a big thank you to John Parfrey for allowing me to use your lovely photograph on the cover.

Thank you especially, to all my students, without whom this book would never have happened.

Recommended Reading

The Alexander Technique Manual by Richard Brennan

Body Learning by Michael Gelb

Ingredients for a Happy Life: Tea, Cake, Meditation by Deborah Coote

Teach Yourself to Meditate by Eric Harrison

Come back to your senses by Jon Kabat-Zinn

Zen Mind, Beginner's Mind by Suzuki Roshi

Useful Information

The find a teacher of the Alexander Technique, visit www.stat.org or www.ateuk.org

Join the National Trust   www.nationaltrust.org.uk

Become a member of Friends of the Earth. www.foe.co.uk

There are many different courses and classes in meditation. Check locally - you'll find the right path for you.

Inspirational and Transformational Books & CDs by Deborah Coote

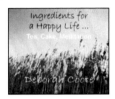

Ingredients for a Happy Life ... Tea, Cake, Meditation

This is a practical, enjoyable and inspirational book covering all aspects of meditation, from why and how to get started, to setting up your own group. It also includes beautiful, creative and useful meditations, inspirational quotations as well as recipes for scrummy 'easy to bake' cakes to share with your meditation group.

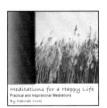

Meditations for a Happy Life Vol 1

This CD contains a collection of transformational and practical meditations taken from the book, **Ingredients for a Happy Life ... Tea, Cake, Meditation** and is suitable for both beginners and those who already meditate regularly. Each track runs for ten minutes and combines guided imagery and analytical meditations to facilitate awareness, well-being and peace.

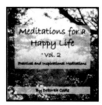

Meditations for a Happy Life Vol.2

This second volume of practical and inspiring meditations contains four extended tracks, lasting up to twenty minutes.

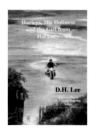

Harleys, His Holiness and the Girl from Hackney by D.H. Lee

'The closest Dan ever got to a spiritual experience was watching Morrisey on Top of the Pops in 1984. Then he meets Kat, the girl from Hackney, and everything changes. Beer, cricket, the mates take a back seat as he steers his life out of the fast lane.'

Based on a true story, *Harleys His Holiness and the Girl from Hackney* is a contemporary, uplifting and humorous account of a journey of transformation.

www.deborahcoote.com